Adulthood in America

Adapting to the Pressures of the 21st Century

Elijah Theodore

TABLE OF CONTENT

INTRODUCTION

Entering adulthood is a transformative trip. In America, this transition is frequently accompanied by unique pressures and prospects shaped by our fast-paced, ever- evolving society. As we navigate the 21st century, youthful grown-ups find themselves at the crossroads of tradition and fustiness, scuffling with new morals, technologies, and societal shifts.

"Adulthood in America: Adapting to the Pressures of

the 21st Century" is a comprehensive book designed to help you understand and manage the complications of ultramodern adult life. Whether you are fresh out of university, starting a career, or just trying to find your footing, this book provides perceptivity and practical strategies to help you thrive.

The book explores the multifaceted aspects of adulthood in four distinct chapters. First, we claw into the prospects and realities that shape our understanding of what it means to be a grown-up today. Next, we'll attack the critical chops necessary for navigating this new terrain, from financial knowledge to time management. In the third chapter, will address the social and emotional confines of adulthood, including erecting meaningful relationships and maintaining internal health. Eventually, we'll look forward, examining how to plan and acclimatize to the ever- changing unborn landscape.

This book combines real-life exemplifications, case

studies, and practical advice to offer a roadmap for successfully navigating adulthood. By the end, you will be equipped with the tools and confidence to not only survive but to flourish in this vital stage of life.

CHAPTER 1

The Changing Landscape of Adulthood

Redefining Adulthood

Gone are the days when majority was marked by a straightforward progression of mileposts similar as finishing academy, securing a job, getting wedded, and buying a house. moment, these labels are frequently delayed, rearranged, or skipped altogether, reflecting the different paths youthful grown-ups take as they forge their individualities. Case Study Jenna's Journey Jenna's story exemplifies the ultramodern redefinition of majority. At 29, Jenna is a successful graphic developer who chose to prioritize her career and particular growth over traditional mileposts. After completing her education, she spent several times traveling and freelancing abroad, only deciding to settle down and consider homeownership after chancing a stable job she loves. Jenna's trip highlights how the paths to majority can benon-linear and acclimatized to individual pretensions and bournes.

The Impact of Technology

Technology has profoundly told how we live, work, and connect, reshaping the geography of majority in unknown ways. From the rise of remote work to the omnipresence of social media, technology offers both openings and challenges for moment's youthful grown-ups. Case Study

Kyle's Remote Work Life
Kyle, a 25- time-old software mastermind, works ever for a tech company grounded in Silicon Valley. The inflexibility of his job allows him to live in a lower- cost area while enjoying a high-paying job. This setup has enabled Kyle to save plutocrat and maintain a better work- life balance. Still, it also brings challenges, similar as maintaining professional connections nearly and dealing with the insulation that can come from working ever. Kyle's experience

underscores the binary-whetted nature of technology's impact on ultramodern majority.

Profitable Realities

Profitable factors play a pivotal part in shaping the experience of majority. Rising living costs, pupil debt, and a competitive job request present significant hurdles for numerous youthful grown-ups trying to establish fiscal independence and stability. Case Study Maria's Financial Struggles Maria, a 26- time-old marketing fellow, graduated with a substantial pupil loan burden. Despite having a full- time job, she finds herself participating an apartment with roommates to manage living charges while diligently working towards paying off her debt. Maria's story is a common bone among her peers, pressing the fiscal complications and strategies numerous youthful grown-ups employ to navigate the profitable realities of ultramodern majority. Social and Cultural Shifts Social and artistic dynamics also impact the path to majority. Changing family structures, evolving gender places, and lesser artistic diversity shape the prospects and gests of youthful grown-ups moment. Case Study Alex's Blended Family Alex, a 32- time-old single parent, navigates the liabilities of raising a child while managing a demanding career. Coming from an amalgamated family background, Alex's experience reflects the inflexibility and rigidity needed to balance the colorful places and liabilities of ultramodern majority. Her trip highlights the significance of support networks and the evolving delineations of family in moment's society.

Conclusion of

Chapter 1

The trip into majority in America is no longer defined by a single set of mileposts or a straightforward path. Rather, it's a dynamic and multifaceted process told by technology, profitable realities, and social and artistic changes. Understanding these rudiments is pivotal for youthful grown-ups as they navigate their unique peregrinations and define what majority means to them in the 21st century.

CHAPTER 2

Essential Skills for

Modern Adulthood

Financial knowledge and Independence

In the ultramodern world, fiscal knowledge is more pivotal than ever.

Understanding how to manage plutocrat, budget effectively, and invest wisely are crucial chops that empower youthful grown-ups to achieve fiscal independence and security.

Case Study David's Budgeting Transformation

David, a 27- time-old design director, realized the significance of budgeting after overspending on unnecessary particulars. He used to swipe his card without important study, chancing himself constantly short on cash towards the end of the month. Determined to take control of his finances, David began using a budgeting app that tracked his charges in real-time. This tool allowed him to see where his plutocrat was going and helped him cut back on gratuitous spending. Over time, David's disciplined approach enabled him to save for a down payment on his first home, illustrating the profound impact of fiscal knowledge on achieving long- term pretensions.

Time Management and Productivity

Effective time operation is essential for balancing the numerous demands of majority, from work and education to particular connections and tone- care. Learning how to prioritize tasks and manage your time efficiently can significantly reduce stress and ameliorate productivity.

Case Study Sarah's Time Management Triumph

Sarah, a 24- time-old graduate pupil, plodded with balancing her coursework, part- time job, and social life. She frequently set up herself overwhelmed by deadlines and unfit to enjoy her free time. Seeking a result, Sarah espoused the time- blocking system, earmarking specific hours to study, work, and relaxation. By sticking to a schedule and breaking tasks into manageable parts, she reduced her stress situations and increased her effectiveness. Sarah's story shows how learning time operation can enhance both academic performance and particular well- being.

Communication and Interpersonal Chops

Strong communication and interpersonal chops are vital for structure and maintaining healthy connections in both particular and professional settings. These chops include active listening, empathy, and the capability to express oneself easily and hypercritically.

Case Study James' Journey to Better Communication

James, a 30- time-old marketing superintendent, set up that poor communication chops were hindering his professional growth. Frequently, he plodded to convey his ideas effectively in meetings, which affected his confidence and performance. Determined to ameliorate, James enrolled in a course on emotional intelligence and communication. Through practice and feedback, he learned to hear further laboriously, express his studies more easily, and understand others' perspectives. These advancements not only enhanced his work connections but also made him a more effective leader, contributing to his career advancement.

Problem- working and Rigidity

The capability to break problems effectively and acclimatize to changing circumstances is pivotal in the fast- paced and frequently changeable geography of ultramodern majority. These chops help individualities navigate challenges and seize openings for growth.

Case Study Emma's Entrepreneurial Rigidity

Emma, a 28- time-old entrepreneur, faced multitudinous challenges while starting her own business, from securing backing to managing operations. Each reversal needed her to suppose critically and find innovative results. When her original marketing strategy failed to attract guests, Emma snappily acclimated by shifting her focus to social media juggernauts, which proved successful. Her adaptability and amenability to learn from failures allowed her business to thrive. Emma's story highlights the significance of problem- working and rigidity in prostrating obstacles and achieving success.

Conclusion of

Chapter 2

Developing essential chops similar as fiscal knowledge, time operation, communication, and problem- solving is abecedarian to navigating the complications of ultramodern majority. These chops not only enhance particular and professional growth but also equip youthful grown-ups to handle the pressures and openings of the 21st century effectively.

CHAPTER 3:

Social and

Emotional

Dimensions of

Adulthood

Building and Maintaining connections

Healthy and probative connections are a foundation of a fulfilling adult life. These connections, whether with family, musketeers, or romantic mates, give emotional support, fellowship, and a sense of belonging.

Case Study Maya's Network of Support

Maya, a 33- time-old schoolteacher, values her close- knit network of musketeers and family. After moving to a new megacity for work, Maya felt insulated and plodded to find her place. Determined to make meaningful connections, she joined original community groups and reached out to associates. Over time, she formed a different group of musketeers who handed support and fellowship. Maya's sweats to cultivate connections amended her life and helped her thrive in her new terrain. Her story demonstrates how laboriously erecting and maintaining connections can produce a strong support system that enhances life's trip.

Navigating

Romantic connections

Romantic connections are a significant aspect of majority, offering fellowship and support. still, they also come with challenges that bear effective communication, collective respect, and trouble to overcome.

Case Study Jack and Emily's Relationship elaboration

Jack and Emily, both in their late twenties, have been together for six times. As they transitioned from council dears to working professionals, their relationship faced new pressures, including managing career demands and particular growth. Through open communication and a commitment to understanding each other's requirements, they navigated these changes successfully. By regularly agitating their pretensions and enterprises, Jack and Emily strengthened their bond and learned to support each other through life's ups and campo. Their trip underscores the significance of communication and collective respect in maintaining a healthy and evolving romantic relationship.

Maintaining Mental Health and Well- Being

Mental health is a pivotal element of overall well-being. The pressures and stresses of ultramodern majority can take a risk on internal health, making it essential to develop strategies for managing and maintaining balance.

Case Study Rachel's Mental Health Journey

Rachel, a 28- time-old accountant, endured significant anxiety and stress due to her demanding job and particular liabilities. Originally, she tried to manage these challenges on her own, but her internal health continued to decline. Feting the need for professional help, Rachel sought remedy and learned ways to manage her anxiety, including awareness and stress operation strategies. By prioritizing her internal health and seeking support, Rachel bettered her overall well- being and recaptured control over her life. Her experience highlights the significance of addressing internal health proactively and seeking help when demanded.

Chancing Purpose and Fulfillment

Chancing purpose and fulfillment is a abecedarian aspect of majority. Whether through career achievements, particular heartstrings, or benefactions to the community, relating what brings meaning to one's life is pivotal for long- term happiness.

Case Study Leo's Quest for Fulfillment

Leo, a 35- time-old mastermind, spent times climbing the commercial graduation, only to feel unfulfilled despite his professional success. Searching for deeper meaning, he decided to pursue his passion for environmental sustainability. Leo transitioned into a part concentrated on developing sustainable technologies and set up a renewed sense of purpose in his work. Also, he started volunteering with original environmental groups, further perfecting his sense of donation and fulfillment. Leo's trip illustrates the transformative power of aligning one's career and life choices with particular values and heartstrings.

Conclusion of

Chapter 3

The social and emotional confines of majority encompass structure and maintaining connections, navigating romantic connections, managing internal health, and chancing purpose. These aspects are integral to a fulfilling adult life, and developing chops to navigate them effectively is essential for particular growth and happiness.

CHAPTER 4

The Future of a Young Adult in a Changing World

Career Planning and Development

Career planning is a nonstop process that involves setting pretensions, acquiring new chops, and conforming to changing job requests. In the 21st century, this process requires inflexibility and a visionary approach to remain competitive and fulfilled.

Case Study Olivia's Career Pivot

Olivia, a 29- time-old marketing specialist, felt stagnant in her current part and sought new challenges. She explored different diligence and discovered a passion for digital health. Olivia took courses to make her chops in this field and networked with professionals in the assiduity. Her visionary sweats paid off when she landed a new job in a digital health company, where she now feels more engaged and agitated about her work. Olivia's story highlights the significance of nonstop literacy and rigidity in navigating career paths.

Lifelong literacy and Skill Development

In a fleetly changing world, lifelong literacy and skill development are pivotal for staying applicable and achieving particular and professional growth. Embracing a mindset of nonstop literacy can open doors to new openings and keep you nimble in the face of change.

Case Study Aaron's Lifelong literacy trip

Aaron, a 40- time-old IT adviser, witnessed significant technological advancements throughout his career. To stay ahead, he constantly pursued fresh instruments and attended shops on arising technologies. Aaron's commitment to lifelong literacy enabled him to remain competitive in his field and handed him with a different skill set that opened new career openings. His trip demonstrates how embracing nonstop literacy can enhance rigidity and professional success.

Financial Planning and Security

Financial planning is essential for achieving long-term stability and security. From saving for withdrawal to managing investments, understanding fiscal principles can help you make informed opinions and prepare for the future.

Case Study Lisa's Financial Planning Success

Lisa, a 35- time-old nanny, honored the significance of fiscal planning beforehand in her career. She consulted with a fiscal counsel and created a plan that included saving for withdrawal, investing in a diversified portfolio, and erecting an exigency fund. Lisa's disciplined approach to fiscal planning handed her with peace of mind and the confidence to pursue her pretensions without fiscal stress. Her story illustrates how visionary fiscal planning can contribute to long- term security and freedom.

Conforming to Change and query

The future is innately uncertain, and the capability to acclimatize to change is pivotal for navigating life's ineluctable ups and campo. Structure adaptability and maintaining a flexible mindset can help you manage query and seize new openings.

Case Study Mark's Adaptability in the Face of Change

Mark, a 32- time-old eatery proprietor, faced significant challenges when the COVID- 19 epidemic megahit. Forced to close his dine- in services, Mark snappily acclimated by rotating to a takeout and delivery model. He also expanded his business by offering online cuisine classes, which came largely popular. Mark's adaptability and rigidity allowed his business to survive and indeed thrive during a period of immense query. His experience highlights the significance of staying flexible and open to new openings in the face of change.

Conclusion of

Chapter 4

Planning for the future involves visionary career development, nonstop literacy, fiscal planning, and the capability to acclimatize to change. By cultivating these chops and strategies, youthful grown-ups can navigate the misgivings of

the 21st century and produce
fulfilling and flexible lives.

CONCLUSION

By understanding the changing landscape, developing essential skills, nurturing social and emotional well-being, and planning for the future, young adults can thrive in the dynamic and evolving world of today. This book equips you with the knowledge and tools to not only survive but to flourish as you embark on your unique journey into adulthood.